Souad Daoud

The colloid cyst of the third ventricle

Souad Daoud

The colloid cyst of the third ventricle

Brain tumors

ScienciaScripts

Imprint

Cover image: www.ingimage.com

This book is a translation from the original published under ISBN 978-620-3-44144-4.

Publisher:
Sciencia Scripts
is a trademark of
Dodo Books Indian Ocean Ltd. and OmniScriptum S.R.L Publishing group
Str. Armeneasca 28/1, office 1, Chisinau MD-2012, Republic of Moldova, Europe
Printed at: see last page
ISBN: 978-620-5-38965-2

THE COLLOID KYSTE OF THE THIRD VENTRICLE

TABLE OF CONTENTS

CHAPTER 1

INTRODUCTION

The colloid cyst is a very rare pathology, affecting only three people per million inhabitants. It is a benign dysembryoplastic tumor (origin poorly defined), represents 0.2 to 2% of brain tumors, and is by far the most frequent lesion of the third ventricle.

It is a tumor mainly of adults in their 30s and 40s, but pediatric cases are reported, and a male predominance is noted [1].

The colloid cyst is a rounded cystic lesion, from a few millimeters to several centimeters for the largest, containing a more or less liquid gelatinous substance. It usually develops in the third ventricle at its antero - superior part, close to the foramen of Monro. A pedunculated and mobile "bell-shaped" cyst with a risk of sudden death. The risk is that as it grows, it blocks the foramen of Monro and at the same time becomes an obstacle to the flow of cerebrospinal fluid. This could lead to hydrocephalus.

Many colloid cysts are asymptomatic and are discovered incidentally.

More rarely, the cyst may rupture. This is why its evolution must be seriously monitored

MRI is the best examination to diagnose this pathology.

The treatment is surgical. The immediate objective is to restore the circulation of the cerebrospinal fluid. This is a delicate surgery requiring a certain technical expertise.

After complete removal of the colloid cyst, the patient is considered cured. Regular monitoring by MRI is prescribed to prevent possible recurrence.

ANATOMICAL REMINDER

ANATOMY OF THE THIRD VENTRICLE :

The third ventricle is a single median cavity deeply buried in the center of the encephalon. Separated from the cerebral hemispheres and seen inside the lateral ventricles, flattened in the transverse direction, it has an average width of 5 mm, a length of 25 mm and a height of 25 mm. The third ventricle is compared to a funnel whose top is inferior, it communicates at the level of its anterosuperior part with the lateral ventricles through the two holes of Monro, and communicates at the level of its posterior part with the fourth ventricle through the aqueduct of Sylvius. Within which one can distinguish: a roof, a floor, an anterior wall, a posterior wall, two lateral walls. (fig.1 ,2)

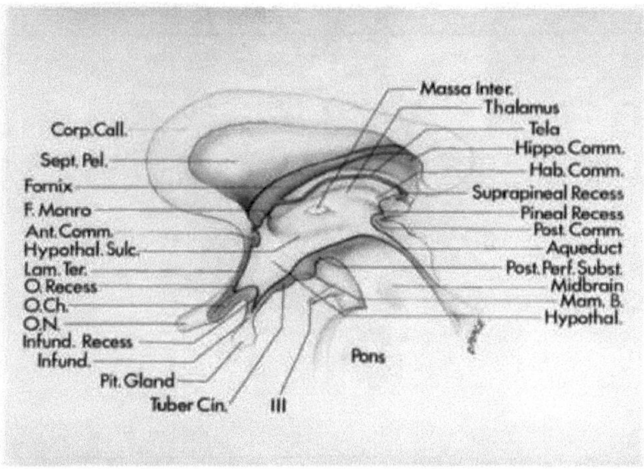

Figure 1. sagittal section of V3, extending from the optic nerves to the aqueduct of Sylvius. Albert L. Rhoton, Jr, M.D. The lateral and third ventricles Neurosurgery 51 [Suppl 1]: 207-271, 2002.

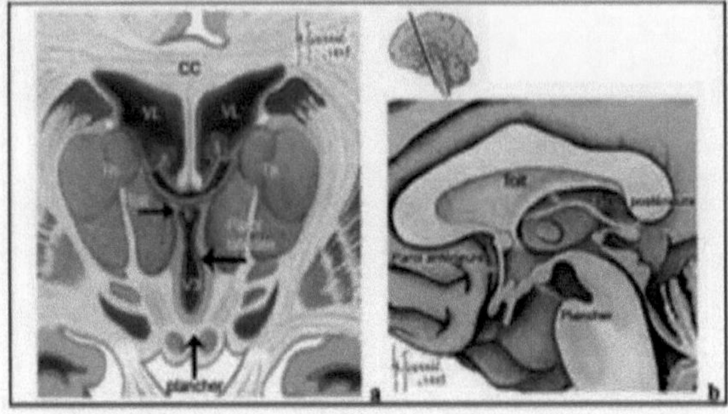

a- Coronal section through the mammary bodies

b- Sagittal section centered on the V3

Figure 2: anatomy of the third ventricle [2]

FRONT WALL : (fig.3)

It extends from the anterior and superior surface of the optic chiasma to the beak of the corpus callosum and is essentially constituted by the terminal lamina (supraoptic lamina). The terminal lamina is a thin layer of gray matter and maggot, attached to the upper part of the chiasma, it stretches upwards to fill the space between the chiasma and the rostrum of the corpus callosum. During endoscopy only the lower two thirds are visible, the upper third being hidden behind the rostrum of the corpus callosum.

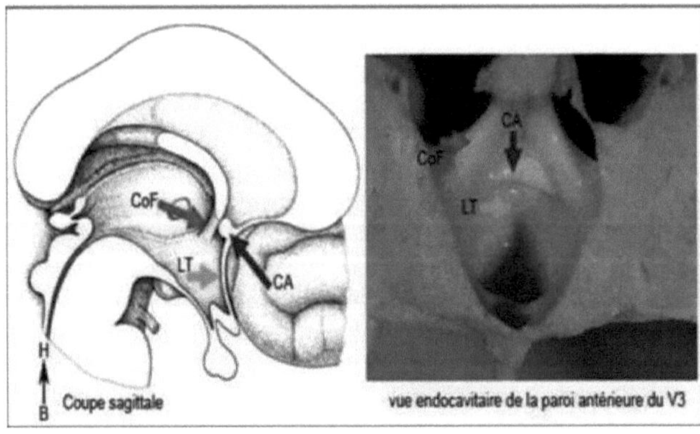

LT= terminal blade - CA= anterior commissure
CoF= fornix column

Figure 3: Anterior wall of the third ventricle. [2]

SIDE WALLS: (fig.4)

The lateral walls of the third ventricle are not visible on an upper view, because they are hidden by the cerebral hemispheres. These walls are formed at their lower parts by the hypothalamus and at their upper parts by the thalamus. The hypothalamic and thalamic surfaces are separated by the hypothalamic sulcus, but the boundaries are often ill-defined and may extend from Monro's foramen to the aqueduct of Sylvius. Under endoscope the lateral walls are shaped like a bird's head. The head is constituted by the internal face of the thalamus, the upper part of the beak is formed by the optic recess, and the lower part by the infundibular recess.

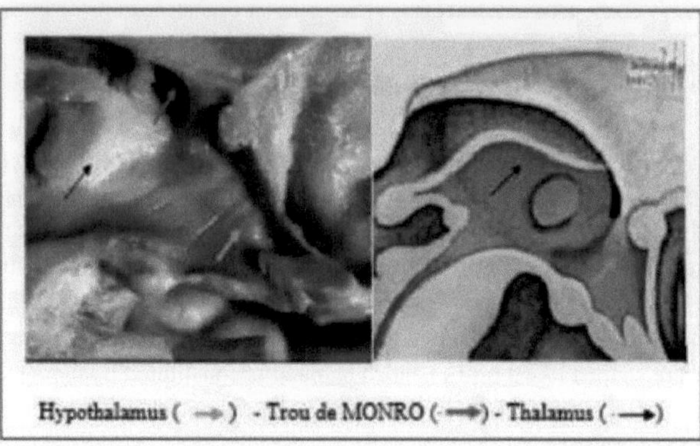

Figure 4: Lateral walls of the third ventricle-sagittal section-[2].

BACK WALL: (fig. 5)

The posterior wall of the third ventricle extends from the supra pineal recess at the top to the aqueduct of Sylvius at the bottom. It is centered by the **pineal gland** (= epiphysis). An anterior view inside the third ventricle from top to bottom shows the supra pineal recess, the habenular commissure, the pineal body and its recess, the posterior commissure and the aqueduct of Sylvius. The supra-pineal recess projects posteriorly between the superior surface of the pineal gland and the inferior part of the choroidal web at the level of the roof of the third ventricle. The pineal gland has two extensions:

- **Superior**: it divides into two bundles of white matter, the left and right **medullary striae** (habenula). They run along the thalamus at the junction of the medial and superior surfaces from back to front. The roof of the third ventricle is stretched between the two medullary striae.

- **Inferior**: it descends towards the superior colliculi (quadrigeminal tubercles). It is crossed by the posterior commissure *(PC), an* interhemispheric commissure overhanging the orifice of the aqueduct of Sylvius. It forms the posterior marker of the bi-commissural line (anterior commissure - posterior commissure), the axis of reference in imaging.

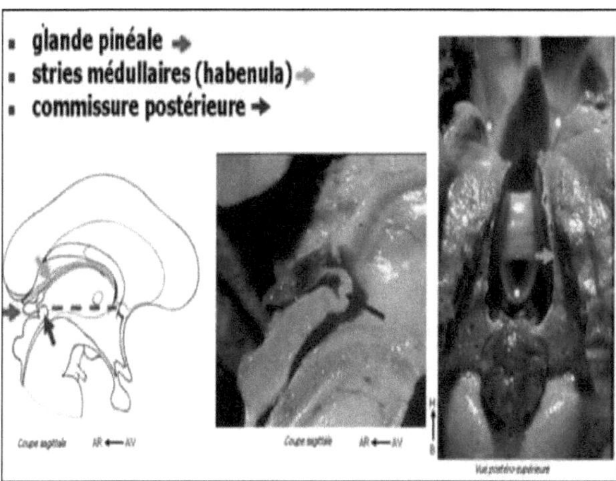

Figure 5: Posterior wall of the third ventricle [2]

THE ROOF : (fig. 6,7)

The roof of the third ventricle forms a slightly ascending arch, extending from Monro's foramen anteriorly to the supra pineal recess posteriorly It is composed of four layers:

- A notch of neural tissue formed by the fornix
- Two thin membranous layers of choroidal tissue
- A vascular layer between the layers of choroidal tissue

The choroid plexuses project parallel from each part of the midline downward at the level of the lower layer of the choroidal web in the upper part of the third ventricle. The velum interpositum is the space between the two layers of the choroidal web at the level of the roof of the third ventricle, this space is usually closed anteriorly just behind the holes of Monro, but it may be open posteriorly between the splenium of the corpus callosum and the pineal body communicating the quadrigeminal cistern with the cistern of the velum interpositum. The lateral part of the roof of the third ventricle is formed by a fissure that extends from the lateral border of the trigone and the superomedian part of the thalamus, called the choroidal fissure. The choroid plexuses of the lateral ventricles are attached along this fissure. During endoscopy, the roof of the third ventricle can be seen in cases of complete or partial agenesis of the septum pellucidum. It appears as a thin, triangular, richly vascularized membrane bordered laterally by the pillars of the fornix [3; 4]

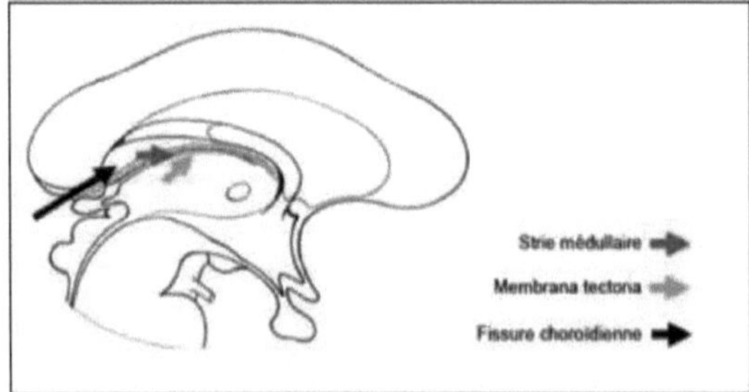

Figure 6: Lateral view of V3. Sagittal section AR<->AV [2]

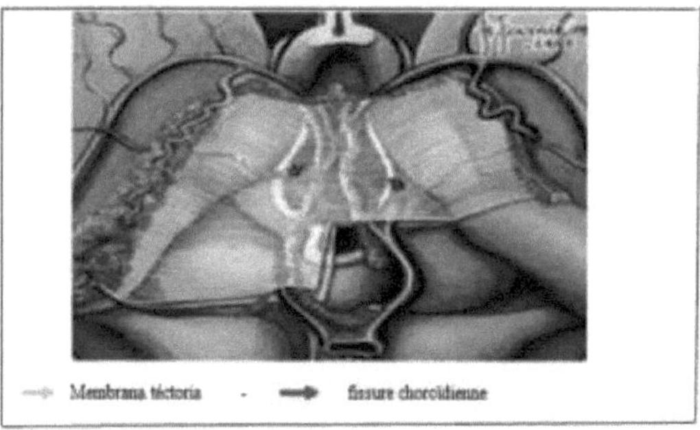

Figure 7: The roof of the third ventricle [2]

FLOOR OF THE THIRD VENTRICLE:

It extends from the optic chiasm in front to the mesencephalic aqueduct in the back. The anterior half is constituted by the diencephalic structures and the posterior half by the mesencephalic structures. (fig. 8)

On the endo-ventricular side, the structures composing the floor are from front to back:

- **The optic chiasm**: appears as a prominence at the anterior border of the floor. It is located at the junction between the floor and the anterior wall of the third ventricle, the lower surface forming the anterior part of the floor, and the upper part forming the lower part of the anterior wall of the third ventricle.
- **The infundibulum of the hypothalamus**: behind and below, a greyish hole, circumscribed by a pink ring corresponds to the infundibular recess.
- **The tuber cinereum**: red parenchymatous structure.
- **the premammillary recess**: translucent zone, sometimes very small but in other cases it can be very large and even deep. Its lower border is considered the safest zone for the realization of the ventriculocisternostomy orifice (VCS); under this recess one can see the termination of the basilar artery and its branches, posterior cerebral artery or even the superior cerebellar artery, especially in case of very advanced hydrocephalus.

➢ **Mamillary bodies**: which form an even prominence on the inner surface of the floor. Classically, they form an acute angle but they can be very distant from each other, sometimes not clearly visible. One of the most important points of reference during endoscopy

> **The posterior perforated substance:** is a depressed space of gray matter, located between the mammillary bodies in front and the medial surface of the cerebral peduncles in the back.

➢ And more posteriorly, the **mesencephalic tegmentum** (central part of the mesencephalon).

➢ The outlet of the aqueduct of Sylvius.

The infundibulum, tuber cinereum, mammillary bodies, and posterior perforated space are located in a space bounded anteriorly and laterally by the chiasma and optic bands, and posteriorly by the cerebral peduncles.

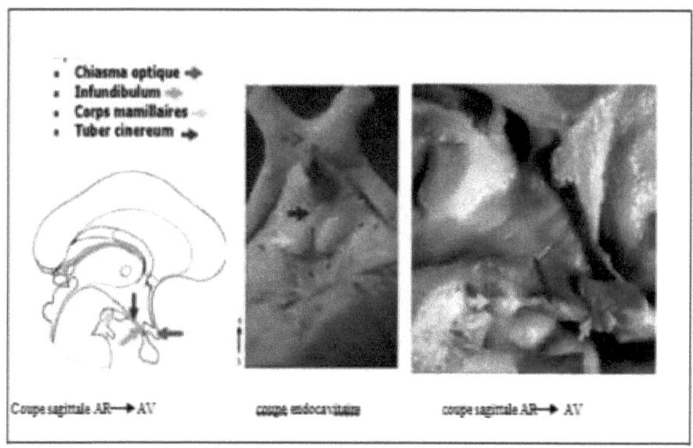

Figure 8: Anatomy of the floor of the third ventricle [2]

- The arterial relationships (fig.9)

Each of the walls of the third ventricle has important arterial relationships, the posterior part of the polygon of Willis and the upper part of the basilar trunk are located below the floor, the anterior part of the polygon of Willis, the anterior cerebral artery and the anterior communicating artery are intimately connected to the anterior wall of the third ventricle, the posterior cerebral artery, the pericallosal artery, the superior cerebellar artery and the posterior choroidal arteries pass adjacent to the posterior wall of the third ventricle.

The anterior and posterior cerebral arteries give branches for the roof of the third ventricle, while the internal carotid, anterior choroidal, posterior cerebral artery, anterior and posterior communicantes give perforating arteries, which vascularize the walls of the third ventricle.

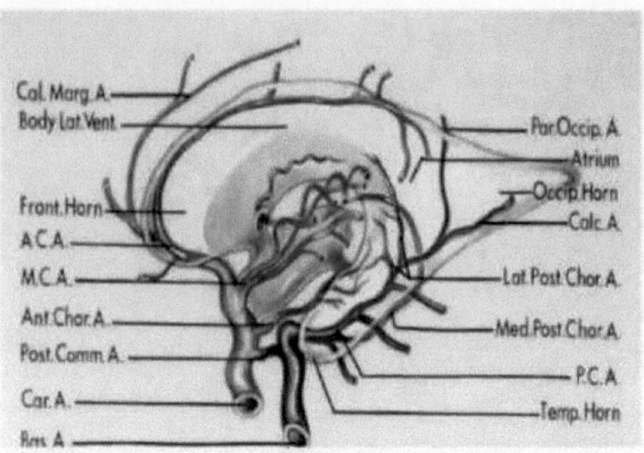

Figure 9: Relationships and arterial vascularization of the ventricles.

Albert L. Rhoton, Jr, M.D. The lateral and third ventricles Neurosurgery 51[Suppl 1]:207-271, 2002.

. - The venous relationships (fig.10)

The venous system is intimately linked to the walls of the third ventricle [5, 6]

The veins draining the deep white and gray substances of the brain, converge into large veins that circulate in and adjacent to the walls of the third ventricle [7]. The veins of the frontal horn, the body of the lateral ventricles and the surrounding gray and white substances drain into the internal cerebral vein; the veins of the temporal horn and the periventricular structures drain into the basilar vein of Rosenthal; the ventricular atrium and the surrounding cerebral structures drain into the basilar vein, the internal cerebral vein and the great vein of Galen.

Veins that collect blood from periventricular structures join to form subependymal ducts in the walls of the lateral ventricles.

These channels are divided into a medial and a lateral group that pass through or adjacent to the choroidal fissure to drain into the internal cerebral vein, basilar vein, or Galen's vein. In the frontal horn, the medial group of venous channels is formed by the anterior septal veins that run along the septum pellucidum and trigone, the lateral group is formed by the anterior caudate veins that run along the ventricular wall of the caudate nucleus. The thalamostriate vein is the largest vein that drains into the internal cerebral vein; it crosses anteriorly and medially the region between the caudate nucleus and the thalamus under the terminal stria, and at the level of Monro's foramen it surrounds the anterior tubercle of the thalamus to join the internal cerebral vein.

Two other veins run along the walls of the third ventricle, the superior and inferior choroidal veins [7]. Both are connected to the choroid plexus of the lateral ventricles and are covered by the ependium, the superior choroidal vein runs along the atrium and the body of the lateral ventricles, and crosses the choroid plexuses. It then drains either into the thalamostriate vein or into the internal cerebral vein next to the foramen magnum. The inferior choroidal vein drains the choroidal plexuses of the temporal horn and the atrium, crosses the roof of the temporal horn downward and forward, and joins the inferior ventricular vein or passes directly into the basilar vein of Rosenthal.

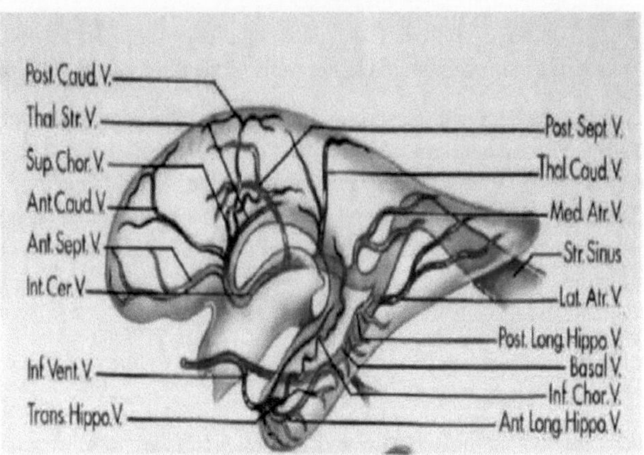

Figure 10: The ventricular venous system.

Albert L. Rhoton, Jr, M.D. The lateral and third ventricles Neurosurgery 51[Suppl 1]:207-271, 2002.

ANATOMICAL RELATIONSHIPS OF THE CYST

The anatomical relationships of this lesion are important to consider, accounting for the difficulties of direct surgical approach. The colloid cyst is closely related primarily to:

- the very anterior part of the third ventricle:

It is usually appended to the ependymal lining of the ventricular cavity, between the two anterior pillars of the trigone, above the anterior white commissure or at the level of the very anterior part of the trigone body.

- Monro's holes:

Monro's holes whose anterior edges are made up of the anterior pillars of the trigone and the posterior edges of the thalamus.

-the choroid plexuses :

The paired and para-medial choroidal plexuses, which run along the arch of the third ventricle and cross the holes of Monro where they continue through the lateral choroidal plexuses.

- deep veins :

The deep veins, constituted by the influxes of the internal cerebral veins that are the septal vein, the thalamostriate vein and the superior choroidal vein. These three tributaries unite just behind the foramen magnum.

These different structures have an essential physiological role, in particular the trigone which is an integral part of the non-olfactory rhinencephalon, and which represents a connection bundle of considerable functional importance between the hippocampus and a whole series of major structures, in particular the mammillary bodies and certain nuclei of the thalamus.

The trigone is one of the elements of the hipocampo-mamillary system that plays a primordial role in the organization of memory. The trigone ensures the fixation of information received by the different cortical systems, which only ensure an immediate retention. A link established temporarily at the cortical level can, thanks to this privileged circuit, become durable. This shows how much a lesion of the trigone can be at the origin of memory disorders of the Korsakovian type. Nevertheless, a purely unilateral lesion can be at the origin of moderate and transitory memory disorders.

CHAPTER 2

EMBRYOLOGY OF COLLOID CYSTS OF THE THIRD VENTRICLE

The colloid cyst or neuroepithelial cyst develops when the neuroepithelium of the roof of the diencephalon invaginates into the third ventricle with the possible consequence of partial sequestration of cystic structures. In most cases, the cyst is intimately attached to the choroid plexuses, in agreement with this theory of the origin of the colloid cyst is the description of neuroepithelial cysts [8, 9, 10].

Surgery in this type of pathology in the anterior and middle part of the 3 rd ventricle should follow the embryological developmental plans of the diencephalic region [11, 12].

PATHOGENY

Colloid cysts have a congenital origin and are classified as dysembryoplastic tumors; pathogenically, two theories are generally accepted:

- The neuroepithelial theory proposed by Shuangshoti [10] explains that the colloid cyst derives embryologically from the neuroepithelium located on the roof of the primitive diencephalon. It is from this epithelium that the choroid plexuses and the paraphysis derive, and he thus attempts to explain the locations along the roof of the V3 of the colloid cyst.

- The endodermal origin is currently the most defended. Hirano [13] suggests that Rathke's pouch cysts, neurenteric cysts and colloid cysts all have an endodermal origin. Morphological studies have shown the possible similarity between the epithelium of these cysts and that of the bronchi and nasal cavities.

Furthermore, Matsushima [14] demonstrated that the ultrastructure of choroid plexuses is different from that of colloid cysts and Rathke's pouch cysts, undermining the neuroepithelial theory.

ANATOMOPATHOLOGY.

The colloid cyst arises in the anterosuperior part of the third ventricle, between the two holes of Monro, posterior to the anterior pillars of the trigone, adhering only to the roof of the third ventricle and to the choroidal web. . It is a well-circumscribed lesion filled with gelatinous fluid.

Macroscopically, it is spherical, oval, smooth with a diameter varying between a few millimeters and several centimeters without parallelism with the clinic. Its color is greenish, grayish or bluish. It contains a colloid, gelatinous or fluid substance.

Histologically, the cyst wall depends on the epithelium of which it is composed; most cysts have a single layer of flattened cuboid cells, which elongates at its base into a thin layer of fibrous connective tissue. This epithelium may be more complex, formed by a pseudo-layered columnar epithelium [15] (Fig. 11).

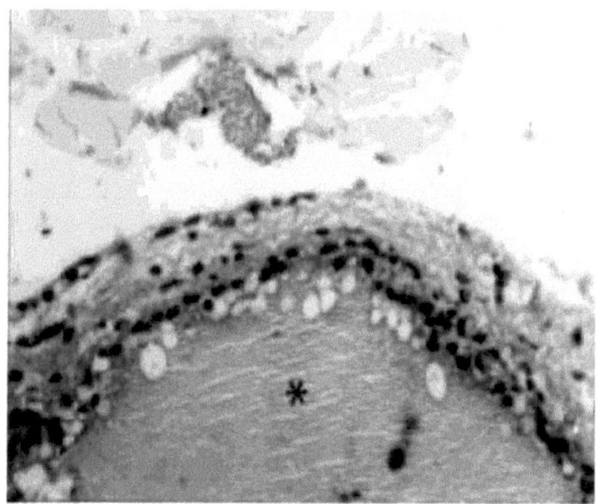

FIGURE 11: Colloid cyst. Wall lined by a layer of columnar cells. The contents of the cyst (star) are coagulated (HPS; X25)

CLINIC

The colloid cyst clinic is characterized by a polymorphism: asymptomatic, latency, sudden death, or symptomatic

The colloid cyst obstructs the holes of Monro and, depending on its size and evolution, it will lead to hydrocephalus, either rapidly or chronically or intermittently, resulting in an intracranial hypertension syndrome evolving in bouts.

Paroxysmal headache is one of the characteristics of colloid cysts; it occurs abruptly when the head position is changed, ceases spontaneously, and may be followed by disorders of consciousness. More rarely, walking disorders are also a characteristic of colloid cysts; isolated or associated with the headache, these disorders may occur in the form of a sudden abduction of the lower limbs or drop-attack, the patient remaining conscious. The "ball valve" mechanism of intermittent obstruction of the holes of Monro by the cyst is a very often put forward explanation, but nevertheless remains controversial, because the intraoperative findings have always found the cyst in a fixed, enclosed and non-mobile position [1].

Epilepsy is a common symptom.

The sudden death syndrome is always sudden but rarely inaugural and a history of cephalalgia is often found. This syndrome is caused by the blockage of the holes of Monro but a compression of the hypothalamic centers [16] or the appearance of a vasogenic pulmonary edema [17] are also evoked.

The incidental finding of a colloid cyst has also been reported.

IMAGING OF THE COLLOID CYST OF THE THIRD VENTRICLE

STANDARD X-RAYS OF THE SKULL

They do not show any specific signs of a colloid cyst

CT SCAN

Examination without contrast medium (thin axial and coronal sections), reveals a hyperdense and homogeneous, spherical or ovoid image located in the anterior part of the third ventricle, adjacent to the holes of Monro in 2/3 of cases. The cyst may be iso or hypo dense [18], the hyperdensity is related to high protein density, squamous secretory activity of the cyst walls, hemosiderin, and microscopic foci of calcifications (Fig. 12). Tumor calcification is not specific to colloid cyst and suggests instead a xanthogranuloma, meningioma, or craniopharyngioma. Injection of contrast medium does not change the density of the cyst, but can sometimes enhance its walls [19].

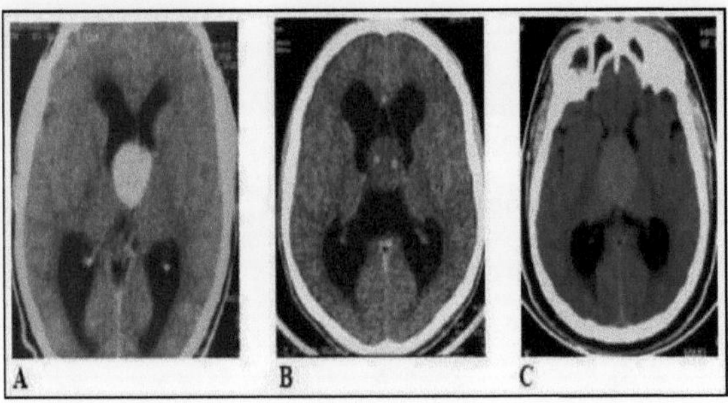

Figure 12: CT scan without contrast medium Colloid cyst;
[A: hyper dense; B: hypo dense; C: iso dense].

MAGNETIC RESONANCE IMAGING

The intensity of the signal at the level of the cyst varies according to its content; in most cases the examination will show a hyper signal in T1, but in T2 it is very intense. In certain large cysts, there may be a hyperintense signal in the periphery with a hypo signal in the center [18].

T1 hyper signal and T2 hypo signal correspond to high cholesterol concentration [18]. T1 and T2 hyper signal corresponds to high protein concentration (Fig. 13).

The appearance of the cyst is heterogeneous on MRI compared to CT. Contrast enhancement of the cyst wall is sometimes reported.

The flow of cerebrospinal fluid on T1 coronal slice examination may be mistaken for the image of a colloid cyst, and axial and sagittal slices correct the diagnosis. Hydrocephalus is frequent and variable; there is no relationship between the size of the cyst and the extent of hydrocephalus. Opening of the septum pellucidum and separation of the posteromedial part of the frontal horns are often found, as well as periventricular edema.

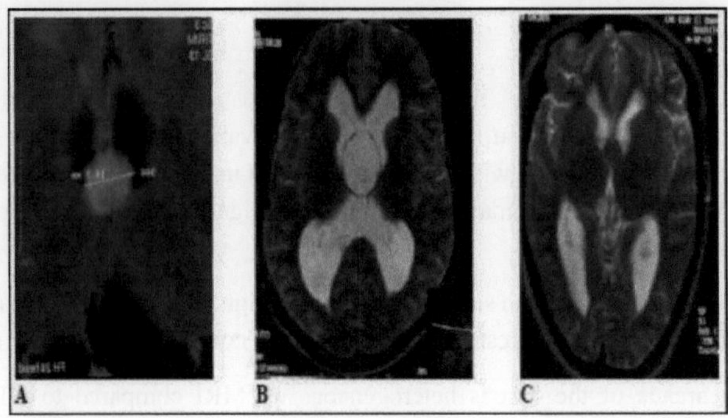

Figure 13: MRI colloid cyst V3; A: in T1 hyper signal; B: in T2 hyper signal; C: in T2 hypo signal

CAROTID ANGIOGRAPHY:

It offers a double interest when a therapeutic procedure is envisaged:

- in order to establish a vascular mapping, in particular of the deep veins.

- in order to eliminate a regional vascular malformation which exceptionally can take certain aspects of colloid cyst, such as an encapsulated arteriovenous aneurysm of the choroidal web.

It should of course be the first radiological investigation during a stereotactic survey.

TREATMENT

The treatment is surgical. The immediate objective is to restore the circulation of the cerebrospinal fluid and to fight against the intra cranial hypertension.

The indication for surgical treatment of a colloid cyst, whatever the method, is not debatable when the revealing symptomatology is one of intra-cranial hypertension. On the other hand, the fortuitous discovery of a colloid cyst, without ventricular dilatation, does not justify a therapeutic procedure.

SURGICAL APPROACHES TO THIRD VENTRICLE

The surgical approach to the third ventricle is classically done through its roof and more particularly through the foramen of Monro. This approach is reserved for lesions located at the level of the upper part of the third ventricle, and uses the transcallous and transfrontal transventricular routes with their transchoroidal and intertriginal variants

(fig. 14).

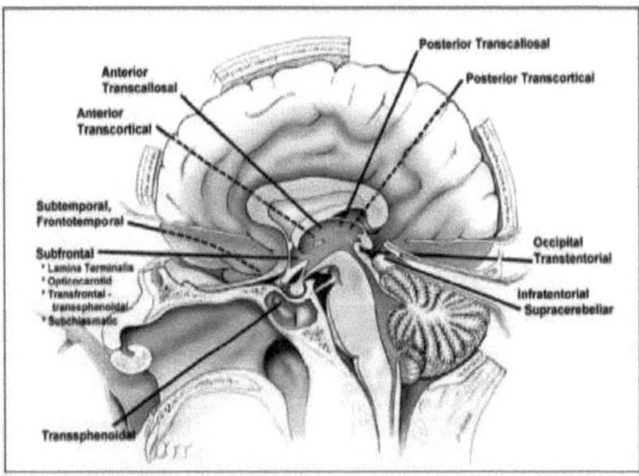

Figure 14: The approaches to the third ventricle; sagittal section exposing the medial tracts along a solid line and the lateral tracts along a dashed line.

Albert l. Rhoton, Jr, M.D. The lateral and third ventricles

neurosurgery 51[suppl 1]:207-271 2002

CHAPTER 3

THERAPEUTIC METHODS

SURGICAL:

The proposed therapeutic methods are surgical. Two types of techniques can be considered

- ☐ direct approach of the cyst and its evacuation, or even its resection:
  - ➢ by simple puncture in stereotactic condition
  - ➢ microsurgical approach (guided by stereotaxis, endoscopy or both)
  - ➢ by transcallous or trans frontal surgical approach.
- ☐ -treatment of ventricular dilatation by shunt.

1/ STEREOTACTIC APPLICATIONS

The application of stereotaxis in third ventricular lesions has grown significantly with the development of imaging and tracking software.

About 15 years ago, stereotactic puncture of colloid cysts was a preferred alternative to open surgery [20]. But it also posed many problems, the first and not least is the difficulty of puncture because of the high viscosity of the colloid substance, not allowing its total aspiration posing the problem of early recurrence [21, 22], The improvement of microsurgical techniques and the evolution of endoscopic methods have supplanted the stereotactic treatment. [20, 23].

2/ ENDOSCOPIC METHODS

Ventricular endoscopy was introduced in neurosurgery in 1910 by Lespinasse, and it is

Dandy in 1918 who used it as a technique to treat communicating hydrocephalus by ablation of the choroid plexuses, then described the ventriculostomy in 1921. From the 1940s onwards, endoscopy was no longer used because of the development of microsurgery techniques and ventricular shunt equipment, and it is only in the last 15 years that neuroendoscopy has been reintroduced, with the improvement of endoscopic equipment, i.e., fiber optics and microsurgical instrumentation.

Ventricular neuroendoscopy has multiple indications and wide fields of action that can be concomitant. Obstructive hydrocephalus is an indication of choice by performing ventriculocisternostomy. Cystic lesions are also treated either by puncture and possibly removal of the cystic wall as in colloid cysts or by fenestration of the cyst walls as in arachnoid cysts. All the fleshy tumors remain, the lesions of the posterior part of the third ventricle are the best example, their biopsy associated with a ventriculocisternostomy has become a common practice; the removal of certain fleshy lesions can also be performed by endoscopic methods.

The use of endoscopic techniques in the surgical treatment of colloid cysts of the third ventricle has taken a great leap forward in recent years thanks to the evolution of endoscopic technology, microsurgical equipment, and the use of laser [24]. The indication for endoscopic treatment of colloid cysts, has become almost superimposable to that of open microsurgery, the significant viscosity or hardness of the colloid substance (hyperdensity on CT) is not a contraindication to this technique as it is for stereotaxis [24]. In certain cases, however, neuroendoscopy is difficult to perform, the main example being the posterior location of the cyst in relation to the foramen of Monro, which makes it difficult to access the neuroendoscopy under the roof of the third ventricle and to dissect the wall of the cyst in relation to the internal cerebral veins and the trigone. There remain all the other situations, of closure of Monro's hole, intraoperative bleeding, and impossible dissection of the cyst wall; in these cases conversion to open surgery is always possible.

The main advantage compared to open microsurgery is to perform the procedure through a drill hole. The approach is the same as that for ventriculocisternostomy, it is often performed under general anesthesia, unless contraindicated. After penetrating the lateral ventricle and identifying the foramen of Monro, a prominent cyst is seen in most classical cases through a dilated foramen of Monro. The cyst wall is often adherent to the choroid plexus, and covered by fine vessels, with the help of bipolar coagulation, the choroid plexus adherent to the cystic wall as well as the tumor vessels are coagulated. The YAG laser can also be used at this stage. The cyst wall is opened with microscissors, and the viscous colloid fluid is aspirated through a cannula with a 10cc syringe; the cyst is emptied, the relaxed cyst wall is coagulated with bipolar or laser, and then cut flush with the micro-scissors. It should be remembered that the traction exerted on the capsule may cause significant bleeding if it adheres to the internal cerebral vein or the thalamostriate vein. Irrigation and possibly coagulation can overcome bleeding from the capsule or the small choroidal arteries, but significant bleeding from the deep veins requires conversion to open surgery. Usually the portion of the adherent cyst posterior to Monro's foramen is always left in place, so as not to cause injury or occlusion of the internal cerebral vein. When the tumor removal is completed, a fenestration of the septum pellucidum is performed at its medial part for 1 to 2 cm, in its thinnest and least vascularized part. The lateral ventricle and the opposite foramen magnum are always explored. Continuous irrigation with saline or Ringer's solution is performed throughout the procedure. The cortotomy is obstructed with spongel. Complications after neuroendoscopic resection of colloid cysts are represented by headache and early postoperative aseptic meningitis, which are related to the passage of the colloid substance into the cerebrospinal fluid [24].

Hydrocephalus

Postoperative problems related to the obstruction of the aqueduct of Sylvius by the colloid substance or by a periaqueductal inflammatory reaction to this substance have been described [24]. Memory disorders related to trigone lesions are also described, as well as epilepsy related to cortotomy [24].

3/ OPEN SURGERY.

3.1) The transventricular transcallous route

The patient is placed in the dorsal position, with the head in the middle, elevated 20°. The incision is bi-coronal and the scalp is lifted forward 6 cm from the coronal suture, which must be highlighted as well as the sagittal.

The bone flap can be either rectangular or triangular with a sagittal base (Fig. 15), exposing more of the midline than the cerebral cortex; the lateral exposure should not exceed 7 cm, and the anteroposterior exposure will have an average length of 7 cm. At the level of the midline, the posterior drill hole is made just behind the junction between the coronal suture and the sagittal suture, flush with the midline, and the most anterior hole is made 7 cm from the first one, still flush with the midline, often this is sufficient, but if there are adhesions of the dura mater with the internal table, an intermediate drill hole is made to better detach them The lateral holes are made parallel to the first two for a rectangular flap, or between the two for a triangular flap at a distance not exceeding 7 cm. In the case of a very large lesion in the third ventricle, with posterior extension, the posterior medial trepan hole can be moved 2 cm posteriorly, knowing that the compromise of the drainage veins posterior to the coronal suture becomes obvious, and the best attitude is rather to lower the patient's head at the time of the operation, to increase the posterior angle of vision under the operating microscope. The use of the Gigli saw is preferred to the craniotome at the midline level as a precautionary measure; most neurosurgeons prefer to expose the superior longitudinal sinus even though there is a risk of injury to it, and ultimately a minimal gain in operative exposure; the other risk of exposing the longitudinal sinus is that during retraction, compression of the sinus is possible resulting in decreased cerebral venous drainage. However, when it becomes necessary to expose the superior longitudinal sinus, it is possible, after having made the bone flap, to gradually remove the bone that covers it with the help of rodents. The dura mater is opened along a para sagittal hinge, and during its retraction one must always be careful not to tear out the cortical drainage veins, because their coagulation and sectioning is only permitted if they are located anterior to the coronal suture and are small in size. The large drainage veins must be preserved, and the preoperative study of these drainage veins on angiography or MRI is always a valuable contribution to the surgical strategy (Fig. 15).

The dura mater must be well stretched at the para sagittal level, but without causing compression on the superior longitudinal sinus, a distance of 3 to 4 cm between the cortex and the scythe of the brain is sufficient for a good exposure.

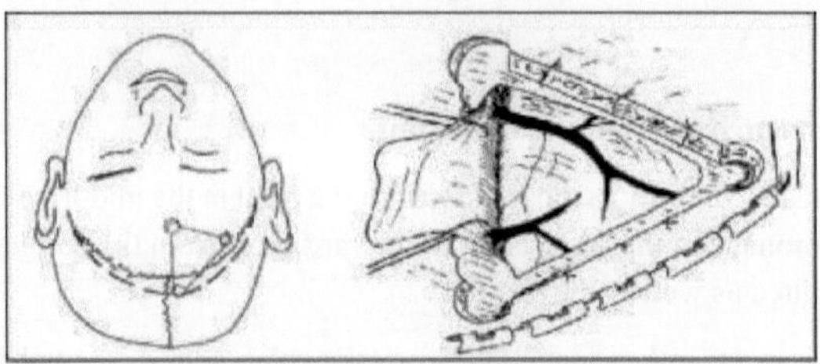

Figure 15 : Anterior transcallous approach, bone flap and dural opening

The simplest landmark that allows to orientate towards the foramen of Monro, is the coronal suture, this one is at the plumb of this hole. Cerebral retraction is performed with a malleable spatula, directed towards the lower part of the scythe, the first artery to be highlighted is the calloso-marginal, it is often located above the cingulate gyrus and can be confused with the pericalleus artery. At this stage a small retraction can be applied on the left hemisphere, which will allow a better interhemispheric dissection, highlighting the corpus callosum which is pearly white in color, while the cingulate gyrus has the gray color of the cortex with a pial vascularization (Fig. 16).

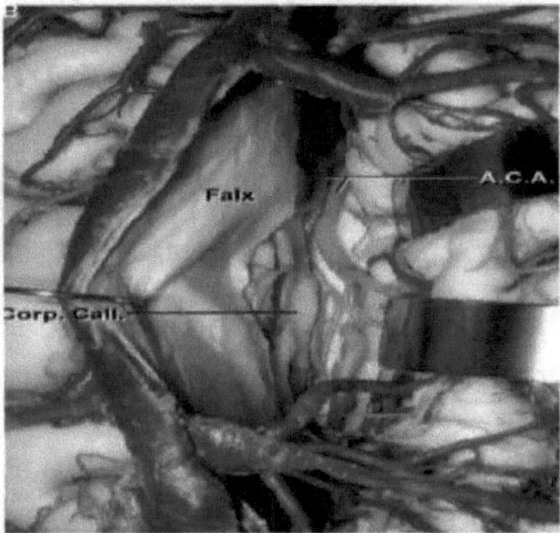

Figure 16: Transcallous approach, interhemispheric stage
exposing the cortical drainage veins, the medial aspect of the frontal lobe and the cingulate gyrus externally, the scythe of the brain medially, and the pericallear arteries, their branches, and the corpus callosum medially.. Albert L. Rhoton Jr, M.D. THE LATERALAND THIRD VENTRICLES Neurosurgery 51[Suppl 1]:207-271. 2002

When ventricular dilatation is significant, the pericallous arteries spread laterally are not always visible, but the corpus callosum is well exposed and allows callosotomy to be performed without the need to highlight them. If both perichondrial arteries are well exposed, it is better to dissect them medially than laterally to avoid damaging their lateral branches. Cerebral retraction should always be gentle and done in alternating fashion to avoid injury especially to the cingulate gyrus. The median callosotomy should not exceed 3 cm (Fig. 17) and is usually performed at the level of the anterior third of the corpus callosum. When there is hydrocephalus, the corpus callosum is very thin and the exposure of the lateral ventricles is easy and quick, but if the ventricles are not dilated the corpus callosum is thick, exceeding one centimeter, and its section is more laborious. The corpus callosum is a vascular body and its division is usually performed with a small dissector, bipolar forceps and gentle aspiration. As soon as the corpus callosum is opened, cerebrospinal fluid flows out under pressure, resulting in cerebral relaxation. The spatula is then placed back into the corpus callosum, lifting the ventricular cavity; the left side of the corpus callosum can be retracted and lifted for better intraventricular visibility, being careful not to achieve compression of the superior longitudinal sinus (Figs. 16 and 17).

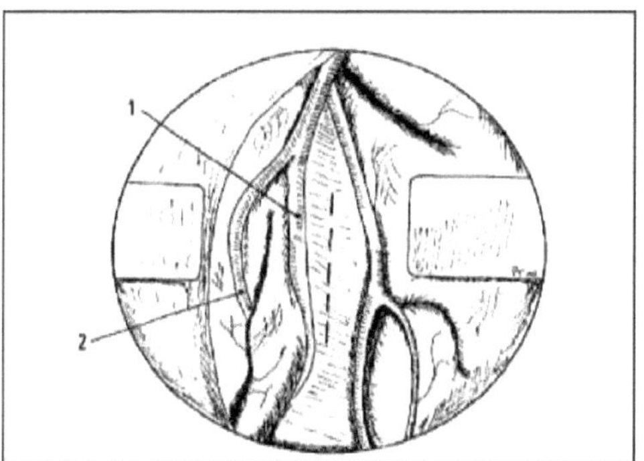

Figure 17: Anterior callosotomy, 1: the pericallear artery,

2: the calloso-marginal artery.

After callosotomy, the right ventricular cavity is exposed and the structures of its floor are identified, namely the choroid plexuses, the septal vein, and the thalamostriate vein (Fig. 18). However, it can happen that one finds oneself unwittingly in the left ventricle and it is then the arrangement of the choroid plexuses in relation to the foramen magnum that will attract attention; it is also possible to find oneself in the cavum of the septum pellucidum where, of course, no anatomical structure of the ventricle is identified. The septum is almost always fenestrated over 1 cm^2 , especially in cases of hydrocephalus or obstruction of a Monro's foramen, otherwise it should be dissected in its thinnest part, avoiding sectioning it near its base. Continuous irrigation with saline is performed throughout the procedure and a thorough lavage is performed at the end of the procedure to remove blood and tumor debris. This approach is sufficient for the removal of lesions in the lateral ventricle, whether or not they extend into the third ventricle, and for lesions developed within the third ventricle, provided that the foramen of Monro is dilated. When these foramen are small or the tumor is large or posteriorly inserted at the level of the roof of the third ventricle, then the inter trigonal approach or the sub- or trans-choroidal approach can be used (Fig. 18).

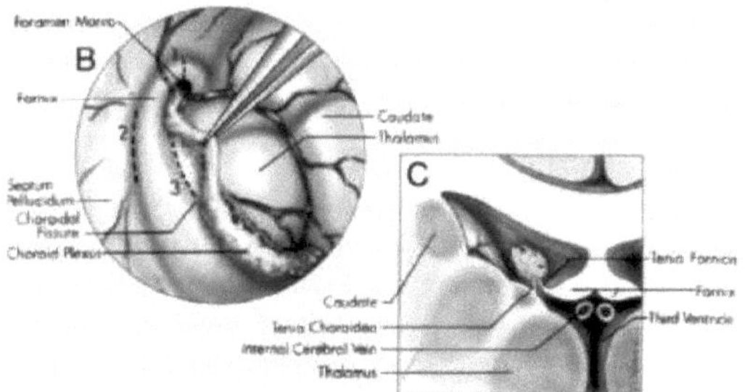

Figure 18: B/ the approaches to the transcallous route; 1= transforaminal with an anterior extension dependent on the anterior pillar of the trigone, 2= the intertrigonal route, 3= the transchoroidal route; C: coronal slice exposing the roof of the V3 and the choroidal fissure with the alternative approaches, transchoroidal, subchoroidal and intertrigonal.

Albert L. Rhoton, Jr, M.D. THE LATERAL AND THIRD VENTRICLES Neurosurgery 51[Suppl 1]:207-271.2002

3.2) The transventricular transcortical route:

The similarities of this approach with the transcallous approach are numerous, from the position, through the bony flap, to the ventricular exploration. The approach is mostly done at the level of the non-dominant hemisphere, except for lesions of the third ventricle which have a strict extension towards the lateral ventricle of the dominant side. The bone flap is rectangular or even square with the same markings as the transcallous flap, the sides measuring 7 to 8 cm, at the midline and it is not necessary to be truly para sagittal (1 cm from the midline) (Fig.19). The cortotomy is performed over 3 to 4 cm at the level of the posteromedial part of the medial frontal gyrus (foot of F2) parallel to the midline (Fig. 19), and the less dilated the ventricles are, the more extensive the cortotomy will be in order to avoid a significant retraction of the cortex. Subsequently, a chimney is made in the white matter until the lateral ventricle is exposed and malleable spatulas 20 to 25 mm wide are placed. The intraventricular approach is the same as for the transcallous route (Fig. 18B). The advantage of the transfrontal approach is to preserve the cortical drainage veins.

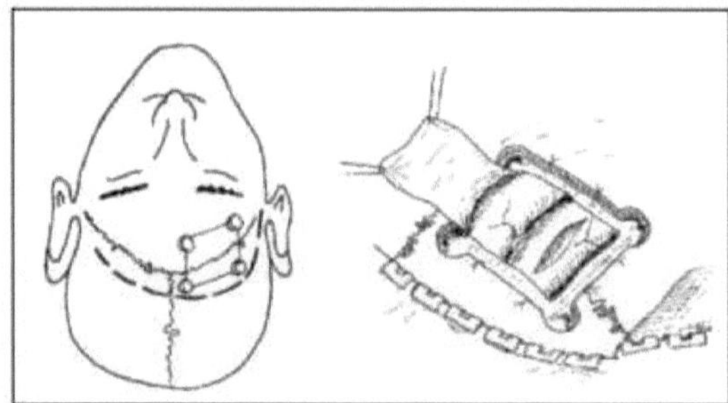

Figure 19 : Transfrontal transventricular approach, bone flap and opening of the dura mater. And cortotomy at the foot of F2.

- The Foraminal stage of the third ventricle

The transcortical approach is valid when the ventricles are dilated and gives a good view of the lateral foramen of Monro ipsi, whereas the contralateral foramen of Monro is rather poorly individualized. In voluminous lesions of the third ventricle, the angle of approach by this route does not always allow good dissection of the lateral walls (Fig. 20). However, this approach may result in postoperative epilepsy or motor deficit when the cortotomy overlaps the motor cortex posterior to the coronal suture or when the retraction is too great leading to edema in this cortex. The transcallous route is an approach used by most

neurosurgeons for lesions of the third ventricle and the problem that remains is the preservation of the cortical drainage veins; the consensus is to preserve the voluminous

veins located next to and posterior to the coronal suture [25]. This route allows multiple viewing angles to explore the third ventricle through Monro's foramen (Fig. 18), with good visibility medially and 10° to 15° laterally [26, 27], especially if the septum pellucidum is removed flush with the trigone (Fig.20) [26, 28, 29, 30, 31]. When Monro's holes are small, over a bulky lesion at the level of the third ventricle, dissection of this lesion is hazardous or even impossible through these narrow foramina. In these cases, the transforaminal approach requires a posterior extension such as the intertrigonal approach [28, 29, 30], the subchoroidal approach [31, 32, 114, 34, 35],
enlargement of the anterior part of Monro's foramen at the level of the anterior pillar of the trigone [30, 36, 37], and section of the thalamostriate vein [31, 32, 33, 34, 35]. In cases where the lesion is small and not visible through the foramen of Monro, the walls of the foramen can be gently spread for exploration of the different parts of the third ventricle, otherwise an extension of the opening of the foramen of Monro can be done by the aforementioned techniques (Fig. 18). Dissection of the lesion at the level of the foramen of Monro must take into consideration several anatomical parameters, first and not least the roof of the third ventricle, whose most important element is the foramen of Monro.

The most important of these is the internal cerebral vein, whose section or interruption leads to diencephalic infarction. Traction on the tumor or cyst can lead to neurovegetative disorders by affecting the medial thalamus or hypothalamus. During exploration of the third ventricle and tumor removal, it is important to avoid traumatizing the trigone medially and the thalamus laterally. Hence the interest in emptying a cystic lesion before dissecting the walls of these lesions adherent to the third ventricle. The section of one or both pillars of the trigone for a better approach and a total excision of the lesions of the third ventricle has been reported by several authors [30, 36, 37, 38], indeed the section of one pillar in case the other one is not destroyed by the tumor does not have serious consequences on the memory but the section of both can lead to cognitive disorders according to the authors [39, 40, 41, 42]. Hemostasis of the tumor bed must always be performed with bipolar coagulation, and it is important to avoid leaving tumor debris or clots in the cavity of the third ventricle, which may lead to obstruction of the aqueduct of Sylvius. There remains the problem of injury to the internal cerebral vein and, to a lesser degree, the thalamostriate vein; in this case, hemostasis should always be attempted with bipolar forceps, trying not to reduce their diameter too much, otherwise hemostatic tissue will be applied to the vascular wound. The principle to remember is continuous irrigation with saline or Ringer's solution.2

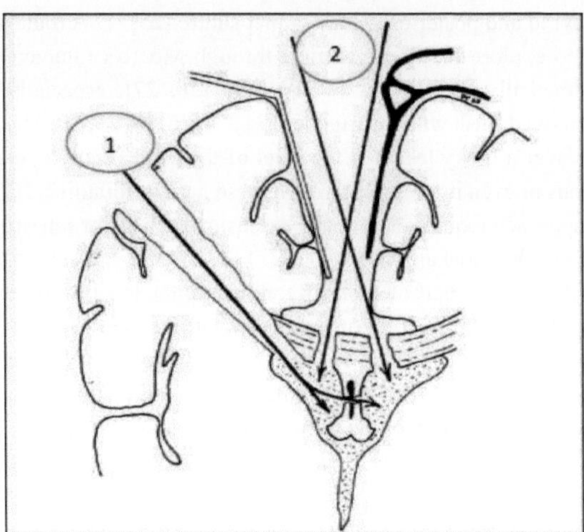

Figure 20: Angulations and directions to the Monro foramens, 1 through the trans frontal transventricular pathway (right), and 2 : through the transcalleuse way in the middle

3.3) The inter trigonal transcallous route

The inter trigonal approach is a complement or a variant of the transcallous approach, which may be chosen as part of the operative strategy (in large tumors of the third ventricle with posterior extension) or used as an alternative when there are difficulties in excision by the transforaminal approach [43]. Edward Busch [44] was the first to publish a description of this technique in 1944, describing the median raphe between the two bodies of the trigone. The operative position and the surgical approach are the same as for the transcallous approach described above (Fig. 18). When the callosotomy is completed under optical magnification, the ependymal surface of the grayish lateral ventricles is identified, as are the ependymal vessels. The first anatomical feature to be highlighted is the attachment of the septum pellucidum to the ependymus (Fig. 21), the structures of the floor of the lateral ventricle are then identified, namely Monro's foramen and the possibilities of foraminal dissection, the septal vein, the septum pellucidum and its relationship with the trigone, the thalamostriate vein, the thalamus, and the head of the caudate nucleus (Fig. 22). Subsequently, the septum pellucidum is fenestrated with the bipolar forceps, flush with the trigone creating a single ventricular cavity. Otherwise, and when there is a cavum between the two septal sheets, transseptal dissection will bring us to the two holes of Monro, as well as the two bodies of the trigone; the inter trigonal raphe must be well identified at the level of the attachment of the septum pellucidum to the dorsal part of the fornix, the inter trigonal incision starts at the level of the two holes of Monro with fine bipolar forceps and a microscopic dissector (fig. 21). This dissection of the trigonal raphe is continued posteriorly for a length of 1 to 2 cm, this limit should not be exceeded, in order to preserve the posterior part of the trigone and particularly the hippocampal commissure, whose damage leads to permanent memory disorders. The size and shape of the trigones are variable, and are often deformed by the expansive process. When the inter-trigonal incision is completed, the tumor appears. The structures of the roof of the third ventricle, namely the choroidal web, choroidal plexuses, internal cerebral veins, and posterior choroidal arteries, may be displaced laterally by the tumor mass.

After aspiration of the cystic contents, the tumor walls are dissected with micro dissectors anteriorly and laterally, where the internal cerebral veins are identified. The floor of the third ventricle and its components will be visualized only when the anterior and inferior tumor portion is removed. Lastly, the posterior portion will remain, which is not always highlighted; its visualization will require an inversion of the position of the head (Trendelenburg), a repositioning of the angles of vision of the operating microscope, and possibly the use of surgical mirrors.

The intertrigonal approach has its limitations, namely small tumors below 1.5 cm in diameter, strictly posterior locations, and lesions of the floor of the third ventricle with predominantly lateral extension [43].

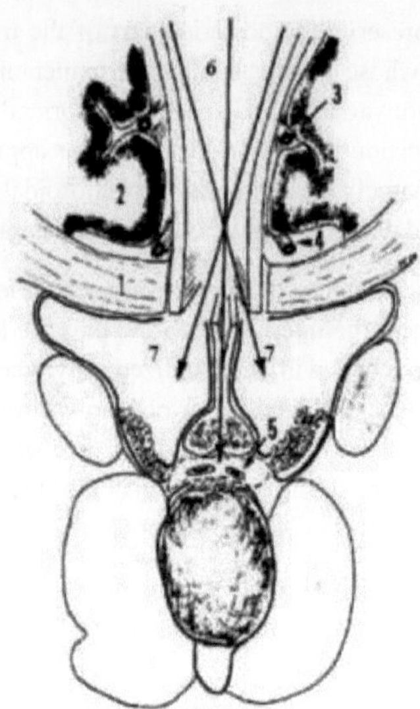

Figure 21 : The anterior transcallous inter trigonal approach allows a trans. Septal (6), and bilateral transforaminal (7). 1 : corpus callosum ; 2 : cingulate gyrus ; 3 : calloso-marginal artery ; 4: pericallear artery; 5: internal cerebral vein.

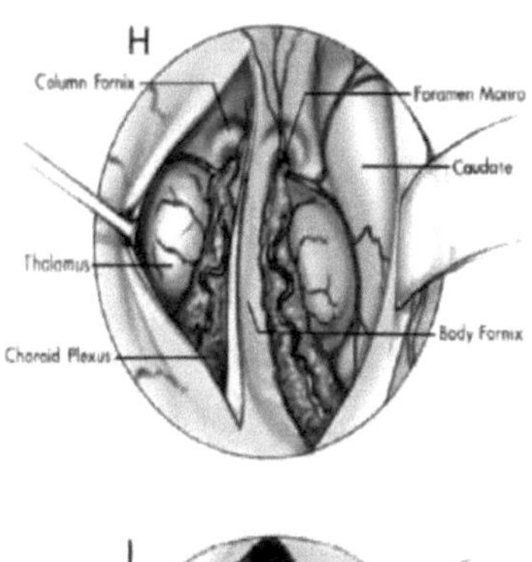

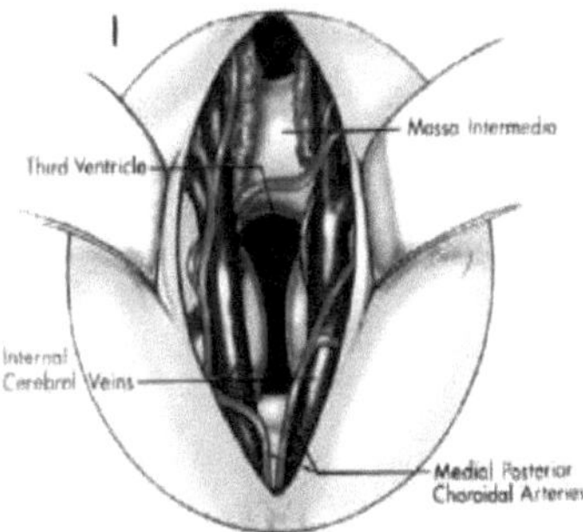

Figure 22 : Intertrigonal approach, H : opening of the septum pellucidum exposing the two VL, the two trigones, the two holes of Monro and the two choroid plexuses; I : opening between the two bodies of the trigone, exposing the V3, the two internal cerebral veins; the posterolateral choroidal arteries and the interthalamic mass. Albert L. Rhoton, Jr, M.D. THE LATERAL AND THIRD VENTRICLES Neurosurgery 51[Suppl 1]:207-271. 2002

THERAPEUTIC STRATEGY

VENTRICULAR BYPASS

Ventriculoperitoneal shunting can be considered as an alternative treatment, whose indication is limited to very fragile patients with significant defects, presenting active hydrocephalus. The complication most often described in this procedure is the derivation of only one ventricle from the other because of the obstruction of the two holes of Monro by the cyst; a contralateral ventricular derivation is then necessary.

STEREOTACTIC ASPIRATION OF THE CYST

Stereotactic aspiration was the therapeutic alternative of choice in the treatment of colloid cysts during the 1970s [20]; the indications are related to the condition of the patient that does not allow an open approach, and to the characteristics of the cyst, which must be of average size between 1 and 2 cm and of a liquid consistency that is not too viscous and allows easy aspiration. The complications of this method are related to poor patient selection; herniation of the rest of the cyst into the third ventricle leading to acute hydrocephalus has
was described by Mathiesen [45], infections, motor and memory deficits, have also been described [46], more rarely vascular lesions of the thalamostriate vein or the internal cerebral vein, have been noted [47].

The postoperative CT scan should look for hydrocephalus, and cystic remnant.

The problems associated with this procedure are the impossibility of puncturing or aspirating the cyst, leading some authors to use spiral needles to cross the cystic wall and larger trocars (2 mm in diameter) to be able to aspirate the contents [20, 23]. Recurrences are not uncommon, and it is therefore reasonable to perform a revision by open surgery or by an endoscopic approach [20].

STEREOTACTIC ASPIRATION WITH ENDOSCOPIC GUIDANCE

Combining the stereotactic procedure with endoscopic visualization is an alternative allowing, in case of problems, the use of endoscopic methods for cyst removal. The results of this procedure are similar to those of endoscopic surgery.

THE ENDOSCOPIC APPROACH

The procedure is described in the chapter on surgical approaches; its results are excellent except for cysts very posterior to the foramen magnum, and in cases where the foramen magnum is closed. Complications are related to injury to the deep veins around the foramen magnum and injury to the trigone.

OPEN SURGERY

The classical transfrontal transventricular approach is used only for anterior cysts associated with ventricular dilatation.

The anterior transcallous approach associated with transforaminal, transchoroidal, subchoroidal or intertrigonal approaches is commonly used for all forms and situations, and for all ventricular sizes; but it is specific for cysts of posterior situation with respect to Monro's hole.

CHAPTER 4

CONCLUSION

The colloid cyst represents 0.2% to 2% of brain tumors. They are more frequent in children than in adults, vary in size from a few millimeters to 9 cm, are spherical or ovoid in shape, have a sessile or pedicle-like main attachment, and sit at the roof of the third ventricle just posterior to the foramen magnum. The choroid plexuses cover and adhere to the upper part of the cyst, whose capsule is covered by a thin ependymal vascularized envelope. The cystic content is very variable, it can be viscous semiliquid, light to dark colored, to gelatinous, more rarely it is of solid consistency. These tumors are rapidly symptomatic because of their early impact on the cerebrospinal fluid flow. The main symptom is HTIC. MRI is the examination of choice for positive diagnosis and precise lesion assessment, on which the therapeutic approach is based.

The colloid cyst is a benign tumor, its therapeutic modalities are multiple, its removal without postoperative morbidity must be the rule.

BIBLIOGRAPHY

[1] . Le Gars D, Lejeune JP, Desenclos C: Tumors of the third ventricle (CM VIII). Neurosurgery. 2000, 46, n° 3 : 296-319.

[2] . HSBOUN D. Morphological anatomy. Faculty of Medicine Pierre and Marie Curie 2007-2008

[3] . DECQ P. Endoçcopic anatomy of the ventricles Pediatric hydrocephalus (Cinalli G., Maixner WJ., Sainte- Rose C.) Springer, Milan, 2004: 351-359.

[4] . RHOTON AL. Jr.The lateral and third ventricles. Neurosurgery 2002; 51 (Suppl 1): 207-271

[5] . DECQ. PH Endoscopy in neurosurgery: the neuroendoscope according to DECQ, 1998.

[6] . LE GARS D, FOULON P: Basic anatomy of the V3. Neurosurgery 2000, 46 n° 3

[7] . NIEUWENHUYS R.: Morphogenesis and general structure in Neuwentheys R (ed) : The central nervous system of vertebrates vol2 Springer Berlin. Heidelberg. New York 1998, 158 -228.

[8] . Antunes JL, Louis KM, Gantia SR: Colloid cysts of the third ventricle. Neurosurgery 1980; 7: 450-455.

[9] . Ciric I, Zivin I: Neuroepithelial cysts of the septum pellucidum. J. Neurosurg. 1975, 43 : 69- 73.

[10] . Shuangshoti S, Robert MP, Netsky MG: Neuroepithelial cysts: pathogenesis and relation to choroid plexus ependyma. Arch. Pathol. Lab Med. 1965; 80: 214-224.

[11] . Bosch DA, Rahn T., Backlund EO: Treatment of colloid cysts of the third ventricle by stereotactic aspiration. Surg. Neurol. 1978, 9: 15 - 8.

[12] . Rhoton AL Jr, Yamamoto. I., Peace DA: Microsurgery of the third ventricle: fact 2, operative approach. Neurosurgery 1981, 8: 357-373.

[13] . Hirano A, Ghatak NR, Wanger JP: The fine structure of colloid cyst of the third ventricle. J. Neuropathol. Exp. Neurol. 1974, 33: 333-341.

[14] . Matshushima T, Fukui MN, Kitawura K. Mixed colloid cysts - Xanthogranuloma of the third ventricle. A light and microscopic electron study. Surg. Neurol 1985, 24: 457-462.

[15] . Aldape KD, Davis RL: Pathological lesions of the third ventricle and adjacent structures. Apuzzo MLJ (2nd ed) Surgery of the third ventricle Williams and Wilkins

1998: 289-315.

[16] .Chan RC, Thompson GB: Third ventricular colloid cysts presenting with acute neurological deterioration. Surg. Neurol. : 1983 : 358-362.

[17] . Findler G, Cotev S: Neurogenis pulmonary oedema associated with colloid cyst in the third ventricle. J. Neurosurg. 1980, 52 : 395-398.

[18] . Zee CS, GO JL, Lefkowitz M, Apuzzo MLJ: Advanced imaging of intraventricular and Para ventricular lesions involving the third ventricle. Surgery of the third ventricle. Apuzzo MLJ 2nd Ed 1998 - Williams and Wilkins Baltimore: 317-368.

[19] . Deramon M, Pruvo JP, Gondry C et al: Imaging of tumors of the third ventricle Neurosurgery 2000; 46: No. 03: 239-256.

[20] . Chen TC, Lavine S, Amar AP et al: Stereotactic. Applications in third ventricular lesions. In Apuzzo MLJ (2nd ed 1998) Surgery of the third ventricle. Williams and Wilkins Baltimore: 847-884.

[21] . Iwasaki K., Kondo A, Takahashi JB: Intraventricular craniophar. : Surg. Neurol. : 38 : 294-301, 1992.

[22] . Yasargil MG, Curcir M., Kis M. and coll, Total removal of craniopharyngioma. JNS 73: 3- 11, 1990.

[23] . Backlund EO: Role of stereotaxy in the management of midline cerebral lesions. In Apuzzo MLJ (2nd Ed) Surgery of the third ventricle 1998: 885-888; Williams and Wilkins.

[24] . Cohen AR, Pereneczky et al: Endoscopy and the management of the third ventricular lesions. In Apuzzo MLJ (2nd Ed) 1998; Williams and Wilkins 889 - 936.

[25] . Ehni G, Ehni BL: Considerations in transforaminal entry. Apuzzo MLJ. Surgery of the third ventricle Williams and Wilkins Baltimore (2nd Ed) 1998: 397-419.

[26] . Harper Rl, Ehni G: The anterior transcallosal approach to brain tumors. Adv Neurosurgery 1979; 7: 9194.

[27] . Villani R, Papagno C, Tomeig, Grimoldin Spagnoli D, Bellol, Transcallosal approach to tumors of the third ventricle. Surgical results and neuropsychological evaluation. J. Neurosurg. SCI 1997; 41: 41-50.

[28] . Apuzzo MLJ, Chikovani OK, Gott PS: Transcallosal interforniceal approaches for lesions affecting the third ventricle: surgical considerations and consequences. Neurosurgery 10: 547-554, 1982.

[29] . Busch E: A new approach for the removal of tumors of the third ventricle. Acta Psychiatr Neurol. Scand 19: 57-60, 1944.

[30] . Dandy WE: Diagnosis, localization and removal of tumors of the third ventricle. Johns Hopkins hosp. Bull. 1922: 188-189.

[31] . Delandsheer JM, Guyot JF, Jomin M., Sherpereel B., Laine E. : Access to V3 by inter thalamotrigonal route. Neurosurgery 1978; 24: 419-421.

[32] . Cossu M, Lubinu F, Orunescu G et al: Subchoroidal approach to the third ventricle microsurgical anatomy. Surg. Neurol 1989; 21: 325-331.

[33] . Hirsch JF, Zouaoui A, Remien D et al: A new surgical approach to the third ventricle with interruption of the striothalamic vein. Acta Neurochirurg. 47 : 135-147, 1979.

[34] . Lavyne MH, Patterson RH J: Subchoroidal trans velum interpositum approach to midthird ventricular tumors. Neurosurgery 12: 86-94: 1983.

[35] . Viale GL, Turtas, : The subchoroid approach o the third ventricle. Surg. Neurol. : 1990 ; 14 : 71-76.

[36] . Little JR, Mac Carty CS, Colloid cysts of the third ventricle. JNS: 1974: 40: 230-235.

[37] . Poppen JL, Reyes V, Horrax C: Colloid cyst of the third ventricle. J. Neurosurg. 1953; 10 : 242-263.

[38] . Le Gars D, Lejeune JP: Introduction and history of third ventricle surgery. Neurosurgery 2000, 46, n°3 : 137-140.

[39] . Batzinski S, Darwar M; Leeds NE et al: Colloid cysts of the third ventricle. Radiology 1974; 112: 327341.

[40] . Eick JJ, Miller KD, Bell KA et al: Computed tomography of deep cerebral venous thrombosis in children. Radiology 1981; 140: 399-402.

[41] . King T, Removal of intraventricular craniopharyngioma through the lamina terminalis. Acta Neurochir (Wien) 1979; 45: 277-286.

[42] . Mac Donald RC, Humphrey RP, Rutka JT, et al: Colloid cysts in children. Pediatri Neurosurg. 1994 ; 20 : 196-177.

[43] . Apuzzo MLJ, Aman AP: Transcallosal interforniceal approach. In Apuzzo MLJ. Surgery of the third ventricle. Williams and Wilkins (2nd edition) 1998 421 - 452.

[44] . Busch E: A new approach for the removal of tumors of the third ventricle. Acta Psychiatr Neurol. Scand 19: 57-60, 1944.

[45] . Mathiesen T. Grane P, Lindquist C; Von Holst H: Third ventricle colloid cysts: a consecutive 12 year series. JNS 86, 5 - 12 January 1997.

[46] . Bosch DA, Rahn T., Backlund EO: Treatment of colloid cysts of the third ventricle by stereotactic aspiration. Surg. Neurol. 1978, 9: 15 - 8.

[47] . Mohadjer M., Teshmar E, Mundinger F: CT Stereotaxic drainage of colloid cysts of third. JNS 67: 220 - 223, 1987.

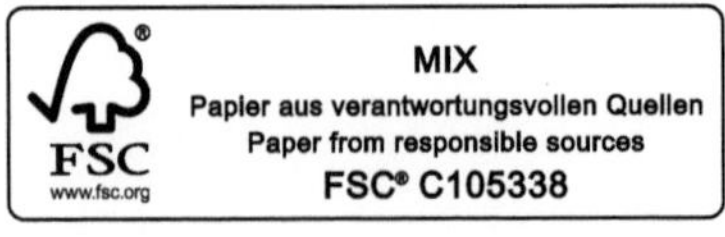

Printed by Books on Demand GmbH, Norderstedt / Germany